CHEMOTHERAPY

Yesterday, To-day, and To-morrow

CHEMOTHERAPY

Yesterday, To-day, and To-morrow

BY

SIR ALEXANDER FLEMING

M.B., F.R.C.S., F.R.C.P., F.R.S.

*Professor of Bacteriology, University of London,
St Mary's Hospital, W.2*

THE LINACRE LECTURE
DELIVERED AT CAMBRIDGE ON
MAY 6, 1946

CAMBRIDGE
AT THE UNIVERSITY PRESS
1946

CAMBRIDGE
UNIVERSITY PRESS

University Printing House, Cambridge CB2 8BS, United Kingdom

Published in the United States of America by Cambridge University Press, New York

Cambridge University Press is part of the University of Cambridge.

It furthers the University's mission by disseminating knowledge in the pursuit of education, learning and research at the highest international levels of excellence.

www.cambridge.org
Information on this title: www.cambridge.org/9781107644656

© Cambridge University Press 1946

First published 1946
Re-issued 2014

A catalogue record for this publication is available from the British Library

ISBN 978-1-107-64465-6 Paperback

CHEMOTHERAPY

YESTERDAY, TO-DAY AND TO-MORROW

———

THE title which I gave for this lecture was too ambitious. It would require a whole series of lectures to do it justice. I must limit it to chemotherapy of bacterial infections, but even that subject is too large for one lecture, so I propose to restrict myself for the most part to chemotherapeutic happenings of which I have first-hand knowledge.

Bacterial infections have existed since time immemorial, and physicians, in all ages, have tried to deal effectively with them. It has been our good fortune to have lived in an era when many of these infections have, for the first time, been brought under control, and there is promise of more advances in the near future.

Until the middle of last century there was practically no knowledge of the bacterial nature of the infections, so before that time everyone was working in the dark, and many and curious were the prescriptions used in the combat against bacterial infections; but we shall get no profit by discussing these.

In the consideration of almost every branch of bacteriology we go back to Pasteur and the latter half of the nineteenth century. Pasteur proved that certain fermentations were due to the action of microbes and that microbes were living objects which did not arise *de novo* from the putrescible material but were descendants of previously existing organisms. Pasteur himself did not do any serious work on chemotherapy, but his earlier bacteriological work stimulated Lister, who had putrefaction of wounds very much at heart, to engage himself on the subject.

There are some who use the word chemotherapy in a very limited sense to cover those methods in which the chemical is administered in such a way that it gets into the blood and attacks the infecting microbes through the circulation in concentrations sufficient to destroy them or modify their growth. This is too narrow a definition, and I shall use chemotherapy to cover any treatment in which a chemical is administered in a manner directly injurious to the microbes infecting the body. In this latter sense antiseptic treatment comes under chemotherapy—call it local chemotherapy if you like. The same general laws govern the treatment whether it is local or systemic, but there are certain particulars in which one has to draw a distinction. There are many chemicals used locally which are so poisonous to the human organism as a whole that they cannot be used for systemic treatment, but large numbers of these, although they had considerable vogue in the past when perhaps there was nothing better, are practically useless as chemotherapeutic agents except in the prophylactic sense. On the other hand, there are some chemicals, e.g. the sulphonamides, which are powerful agents for systemic treatment but which are frequently of little use when locally applied to a suppurating area, as their action is neutralized by substances occurring in the pus.

If a chemical is to be effective in the treatment of established infection it is necessary that, in addition to killing or inhibiting the growth of the microbes on the surface, it should be able to diffuse into the tissues to reach the microbes there. In a septic wound there are, of course, microbes in the cavity of the wound, but far more important are those which have invaded the walls.

Lister, like all other surgeons of 90 years ago, was struggling with the problem of septic wounds. To him, Pasteur's work came as a ray of light in the darkness. Putrefaction was due to living microbes which were introduced from outside. He set to work to prevent them being introduced.

7

He cleansed his hands and his instruments, and treated them with chemicals, and he used a carbolic spray to kill bacteria in the air and prevent them reaching his operation wounds. In this way he revolutionized surgery.

That was prophylactic chemotherapy. Lister himself recognized that carbolic acid, which was his standby as an antiseptic, was very poisonous to the tissues. There are times, however, when if it is possible to kill all the bacteria in an infected area with a chemical it may be worth while to sacrifice certain tissues locally, but the usefulness of such toxic chemicals is very strictly limited.

As a result of the success of Lister's antiseptic treatment a large variety of chemicals were introduced as local chemotherapeutic agents for the treatment of localized infections. In time bacteriology was put on a sound basis, and the antibacterial effect of these chemicals could be tested in the laboratory. In the early days of the laboratory investigation of these antiseptics (or local chemotherapeutic agents) little attention was paid to anything but their action on bacteria in a watery medium. This resulted in very high values being given to substances like mercuric chloride, which could be diluted about half a million times before it lost its power of inhibiting the growth of bacteria when tested in watery medium, but which was largely 'quenched' in the presence of serum or blood.

But none of these chemicals had much effect in destroying bacteria once they had invaded the tissues. I commenced medicine in the early years of this century. Then Lister's methods were rather discredited—asepsis had taken the place of antiseptics for prophylactic chemotherapy, but for the treatment of infections which were already established, a great variety of chemicals were used. Carbolic acid, boric acid, mercuric chloride, silver salts, iodine, etc., were used extensively on septic conditions, but there did not in most cases appear to be any striking benefit except perhaps in some superficial infections. These chemicals were used quite empirically and were, I suppose, a relic of the antiseptic days when they had proved valuable in prophylaxis. They failed in treatment. They were either non-diffusible, or if they were diffusible they poisoned the tissues more than the bacteria. One of the first things I learnt in the casualty room was not to put a carbolic compress on a septic finger or carbolic gangrene was likely to result.

Then came the war of 1914–18. The aseptic surgeons were suddenly presented with masses of wounds, all of which became infected. The primary infection was from the soil and the soldiers' clothing and was largely anaerobic, but after a week or

9

more in hospital this was replaced by the usual septic infection of civil life—mainly staphylococci, streptococci and coliform and diphtheroid bacilli.

Into these wounds all manner of chemicals were poured in an attempt to destroy the infecting microbes. It was not so difficult sometimes to get rid of the majority of the microbes in the cavity of the wound—they could for the most part be washed out by simple irrigation with normal saline—but none of the chemicals had much action on the bacteria in the infected wound walls.

I might here show you a simple experiment which illustrated the inability of chemicals to sterilize even the cavity of a wound. From a test-tube some small processes were drawn to imitate the irregular processes in the cavity of a war wound. The tube was now filled with serum and infected with the usual bacteria which were found in wounds. Here we had an irregular infected cavity, but there was no possibility of the microbes invading the walls (Fig. 1). The 'artificial wound' was 'dressed' by inverting the

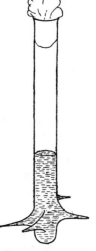

Fig. 1. Artificial wound.

tube and allowing the fluid to escape. This was replaced with an antiseptic which was allowed to remain in the tube for various times up to 24 hours, after which it was poured out and replaced by serum. The tube was then incubated, and next day there was a copious growth of bacteria with all the chemical antiseptics tested. The antiseptic had been unable to diffuse into the processes and kill the bacteria there, so as soon as the antiseptic was removed they grew out again and contaminated the whole tube.

Another observation made in the 1914–18 war is of some importance in local chemotherapy. In 1917 probably the most favoured method of treatment of a septic wound was the Carrell Dakin treatment. Dakin's fluid (sodium hypochlorite) was instilled into a wound every 2 hours. I had an opportunity of studying the length of time that Dakin's fluid remained active in a wound; I found a cup-shaped wound into which I could put a fluid and withdraw the whole of it after any interval. When Dakin's fluid was left in such a wound for 10 minutes its potency had diminished below the limit at which it was antiseptic in serum. It followed from this that for 1 hour and 50 minutes out of every 2 hours there was no effective chemical antiseptic in the wound. But Dakin's fluid had another quite unexpected action. After it had been applied it caused a marked increase in the transudation of fluid from the walls of the wound which persisted for some time after fluid was removed.

Fig. 2 illustrates this increased transudation. Incidentally the number of living bacteria was not

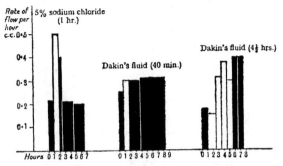

Fig. 2. Increased transudation. Dakin's fluid. Black columns = before and after. White columns = during application.

reduced in the exudate after the application of Dakin's fluid for $4\frac{1}{2}$ hours.

I suggest that the chief virtue of Dakin's fluid was not direct antiseptic action, but that it lay in this power of stimulating the exudation of fluid from the infected walls of the wound, thus draining the oedematous tissues just as did hypertonic saline solution, which was another favourite dressing for a septic wound. But Dakin's fluid *in vitro* in the

12

absence of serum or pus was a powerful anti-bacterial agent, so all its benefits in treatment were ascribed to its direct antiseptic action.

It is desirable in the investigation of the action of these chemicals to see how long they remain active in the body, and before we class them as chemotherapeutic agents we should see if possible whether the apparently beneficial effect is due to a direct antibacterial action.

I have said that Lister recognized the local toxic action of his favourite antiseptic, carbolic acid, but the toxic action of many of its successors was not so obvious and was sometimes forgotten.

Later, and especially in the war of 1914–18, some notice was taken of the action of these chemicals on cells and especially on leucocytes, as it was not difficult to test the effect of a chemical on leucocytic function. Most usually it was the phagocytic power of the leucocytes which was tested, but the methods adopted did not always give a true picture. The effect of the chemical on bacteria was tested by its power to inhibit growth and its effect on leucocytes by its power to inhibit phagocytosis. This at first sight seems a perfectly good method, but actually the chemical acts on the bacteria during a period of hours, whereas in the phagocytic experiments the maximum time of action was 15 minutes. When blood is mixed with bacteria phagocytosis takes place very rapidly, and even in 5 minutes the cells will take up large numbers of microbes. That being so, if a chemical is added to the mixture which does not have a *rapid* lethal action on the leucocyte the latter continues to phagocyte the bacteria, and if the observation is ended after 15 minutes quite a false idea is obtained as to the destructive action of the chemical on the leucocyte. Acriflavine is a good example of this. It is a slow-acting bactericidal and leucocidal agent. If its antileucocytic power is tested only for 15 minutes it has been found that it requires a dilution of 1 in 500 to reduce the amount of phagocytosis by 50 %. If, however, the chemical is allowed to remain in contact with the blood for 5 hours before the phagocytic test is made, it is found that a 1 in 500,000 dilution will cause a 50 % reduction in the amount of phago-cytosis. As it takes a 1 in 200,000 dilution to in-hibit the growth of bacteria the 'Therapeutic index' calculated after 15 minutes' exposure of leucocytes is 400, whereas if the time of exposure had been 5 hours (a more reasonable time) it would have been 0·4—a considerable difference.

In 1924 I adapted Wright's slide-cell method to show in one experiment the action of chemicals on bacteria and on leucocytes. Dilutions of the chemical were made in normal saline, and to these was added an equal volume of human blood suitably infected with the test bacteria (staphylococci or streptococci). These mixtures were run into slide cells, sealed and incubated.* Normal human blood kills off about 95 % of the bacteria, but if the leucocytes are removed the bactericidal power disappears. In the case of all the chemical antiseptics in use there was a range of concentration where the chemical destroyed the leucocytes without interfering with the growth of the bacteria. This destruction of the leucocytes removed the natural antibacterial power of the blood, and resulted in an increased growth of the bacteria. This I regard as the most important series of experiments I have ever done, and it had a certain bearing on more recent advances of which I shall speak later.

Fig. 3 shows the result obtained with carbolic acid. There is an antileucocytic zone of concentration resulting in increased growth of the bacteria, and at a concentration of 1 in 640 the bactericidal power of the blood is completely destroyed and every microbe grows.

Let us now come to chemotherapy in the narrower sense, i.e. the attack on the infective microbe through the circulation.

* With slow-acting antiseptics the chemical was mixed with the blood and allowed to stand for a suitable interval, after which the bacteria were added and the mixture incubated.

There was the mercury treatment of syphilis. Mercury was swallowed, injected or rubbed into the skin. There were no tests proving that it ever reached the circulation in concentrations inimical to the spirochaete, but from the clinical results

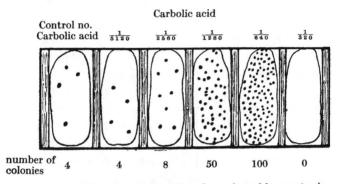

Fig. 3. Effect of carbolic acid on bacteria and leucocytes in human blood.

we may presume that something happened after a strenuous course of mercury which influenced the disease. With no more evidence we might assume that potassium iodide had some direct action on the infective agent of syphilis, actinomycosis and other diseases.

In the early days of antiseptics it was shown that formalin inhibited the growth of the tubercle bacillus in quite high dilution. An eminent physician in the days of my youth recommended that formalin should be injected intravenously for the treatment of tubercle. I should like to show what happens when formalin is added to blood infected with *Staphylococcus*, an organism at least as susceptible to its action as is the tubercle bacillus.

The experiment is similar to the one I have already described with carbolic acid and the result is much the same; there is a range of concentration which encourages growth by destroying the leuco-cytes. Actually the amount administered was very much less than that necessary to influence the growth of the bacteria in any way. It was fortu-nate, perhaps, that sufficient of the chemical could not be injected to destroy the leucocytes (Fig. 4 A).

Exactly the same may be said of quinine, which was recommended as an injection for the treatment of streptococcal septicaemia (Fig. 4 B).

Eusol, too, was recommended in 1915 as an intravenous injection for *Streptococcus* septicaemia. I show you the result of mixing Eusol with infected human blood (Fig. 4 C). If several litres could have been injected the leucocytes would have suffered, but fortunately that was not possible.

Mercuric chloride has been recommended as an intravenous injection for streptococcal septicaemia. This is more interesting. When it is tested with *Staphylococcus* it gives a result similar to those

17

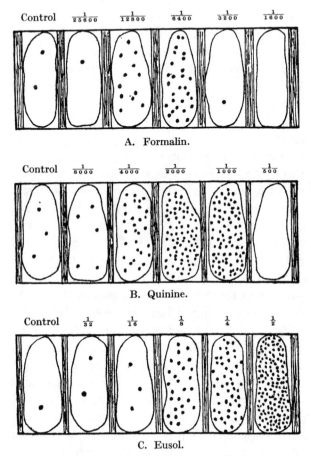

| Control | $\frac{1}{25600}$ | $\frac{1}{12800}$ | $\frac{1}{6400}$ | $\frac{1}{3200}$ | $\frac{1}{1600}$ |

A. Formalin.

| Control | $\frac{1}{8000}$ | $\frac{1}{4000}$ | $\frac{1}{2000}$ | $\frac{1}{1000}$ | $\frac{1}{500}$ |

B. Quinine.

| Control | $\frac{1}{32}$ | $\frac{1}{16}$ | $\frac{1}{8}$ | $\frac{1}{4}$ | $\frac{1}{2}$ |

C. Eusol.

Fig. 4. Effect of chemicals on the bactericidal power of
human blood.

Black spots represent bacterial colonies.

18

quoted above, but when *Streptococcus pyogenes* is used as the test organism an extraordinary result is obtained (Fig. 5). Here 1/20,000 destroys leucocytic action and allows the streptococci to grow, but weaker dilutions completely stop growth of the streptococci—but only if the leucocytes are present. The leucocytes cannot do this by themselves (vide control) nor can the mercuric chloride (vide 1/20,000 cell), but in some way the combined effect of the two can completely inhibit growth. If conditions are carefully adjusted this inhibitory effect can be seen with a dilution of almost 1 in half a million—a quantity which can almost be reached by a therapeutic dose of the drug.

Scientific chemotherapy dates from Ehrlich and scientific chemotherapy of a bacterial disease from Ehrlich's Salvarsan, which in 1910 revolutionized the treatment of syphilis. The story of Salvarsan has often been told, and I need not go further into it except to say that it was the first real success in the chemotherapeutic treatment of a bacterial disease. Ehrlich originally aimed at 'Therapia magna sterilisans', which can be explained as a blitz sufficient to destroy at once all the infecting microbes. This idea was not quite realized, and now the treatment of syphilis with arsenical preparations is a long-drawn-out affair. But it was extraordinarily successful treatment, and stimulated

19

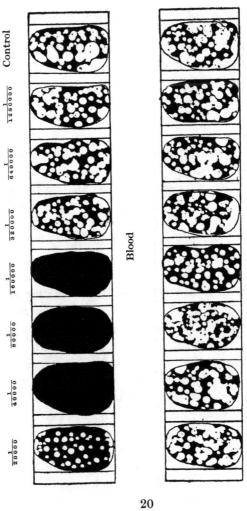

Fig. 5. Action of mercuric chloride on haemolytic streptococci in blood.

work on further chemotherapeutic drugs. While they had success in some parasitic diseases the ordinary bacteria which infect us were still unaffected.

Some aniline dyes were shown by Churchman many years ago to have remarkable selective properties as antibacterial agents, and they became prominent as antiseptics in septic wounds after Browning in 1917 described the action of acriflavine. This substance has been recommended as a chemotherapeutic agent for intravenous injection, but it proved to have some toxicity for the liver. When it is injected it very rapidly disappears from the blood and all the tissues are stained except the nervous system. The following figures give the antibacterial power of the blood before and at intervals after an intravenous injection of acriflavine, and these are contrasted with the result obtained after an intravenous injection of hypertonic sodium chloride:

Bactericidal power of blood after intravenous injection (in rabbit)

A. Acriflavine		B. NaCl	
20 c.c. of 1/1000		3 c.c. of 10%	
	No. of colonies		No. of colonies
Before injection	87	Before	25
1 min. after injection	62	2 min. after	28
3 min. after injection	87	30 min. after	8
45 min. after injection	92	2 hr. after	0
		6 hr. after	0

Whereas the increased antibacterial power after acriflavine was slight and evanescent, there was a very considerable increase after sodium chloride which lasted for hours. This could not be due directly to the sodium chloride, which in itself was not antibacterial, and the only change that could be discovered was some rise in the opsonic power of the serum. This could not be true chemotherapy, but it illustrates another of the factors which have to be borne in mind in the investigation of the action of these drugs.

Then Sanocrysin was introduced as a chemotherapeutic agent against the tubercle bacillus, and it was said that after administration so many tubercle bacilli were destroyed that an antitubercular serum had to be given to prevent poisoning with the toxins of the dead bacilli. This was another failure; Fry showed that Sanocrysin in the concentrations used had no action on the growth of the tubercle bacillus, but it is still used for the treatment of tuberculosis, although it is not with the idea of direct chemotherapeutic action.

Long before this it had been noticed that some microbes were antagonistic to others—Pasteur himself was the first to show this—and some microbic substances or antibiotics had been used for local treatment for their direct effect on the infection. Notable among these was pyocyanase —a product of *B. pyocyaneus*—which was introduced early in the century. It was not very successful and fell into disuse.

I have said something of what happened in the past—let us say up to 10 years ago. That was yesterday.

Now we have to go on to a consideration of the chemotherapeutic happenings of to-day, and by to-day I mean the last decade. Things have moved indeed, and it is safe to say that in the last ten years more advances have been made in the chemotherapy of bacterial infections than in the whole history of medicine.

TO-DAY

It was in 1932 that a sulphonamide of the dye chrysoidine was prepared, and in 1935 Domagk showed that this compound (Prontosil) had a curative action on mice infected with streptococci. It was only in 1936, however, that its extraordinary clinical action in streptococcal septicaemia in man was brought out. Thus just 10 years ago and 26 years after Ehrlich had made history by producing Salvarsan, the medical world woke up to find another drug which controlled a bacterial disease. Not a venereal disease this time, but a common septic infection which unfortunately not infre-

23

quently supervened in one of the necessary events of life—childbirth.

Before the announcement of the merits of the drug, Prontosil, the industrialists concerned had perfected their preparations and patents. Fortunately for the world, however, Tréfouel and his colleagues in Paris soon showed that Prontosil acted by being broken up in the body with the liberation of sulphanilamide, and this simple drug, on which there were no patents, would do all that Prontosil could do. Sulphanilamide affected streptococcal, gonococcal and meningococcal infections as well as *B. coli* infections in the urinary tract, but it was too weak to deal with infections due to organisms like pneumococci and staphylococci.

Two years later Ewins produced sulphapyridine —another drug of the same series—and Whitby showed that this was powerful enough to deal with pneumococcal infections. This again created a great stir, for pneumonia is a condition which may come to every home.

The hunt was now on and chemists everywhere were preparing new sulphonamides—sulphathiazole appeared, which was still more powerful on streptococci and pneumococci than its predecessors, and which could clinically affect generalized staphylococcal infections.

Since then we have had sulphadiazine, sulpha-merazine, sulphamethazine and others. But of these we need not go into detail, so much has already been written about them. Meantime there had appeared other sulphonamide compounds, such as sulphaguanidine, which were not absorbed from the alimentary tract, and these were used for the treatment of intestinal infections like dysentery.

The sulphonamides were very convenient for practice, in that they could be taken by the mouth. The drug was absorbed into the blood, where it appeared in concentration more than was necessary to inhibit the growth of sensitive bacteria. From the blood it could pass with ease into the spinal fluid, so it was eminently suited for the treatment of cerebrospinal infections. The sulphonamides were excreted in high concentration in the urine, so that although they were unable to control generalized infections with coliform bacilli they rapidly eliminated similar infections of the urinary tract. In contrast to the older antiseptics they had practically no toxic action on the leucocytes. There were disadvantages in that they were not without toxicity to the patient. Many suffered from nausea and vomiting, in some the bone marrow was affected with resultant agranulo-cytosis, and in others the drug was excreted in such a concentration that it crystallized out in the kidney tubules with serious results.

However, for the first time we had something which did control many common bacterial infections.

It was found, however, that the action was inhibited by certain substances. Early in the work on sulphanilamide it was noticed that, *in vitro*, complete bacteriostasis was obtained with a small inoculum, while if the inoculum was large the microbes grew freely. Plate I illustrates this clearly.

It was shown that haemolytic streptococci, one of the most sensitive organisms, contained a substance which inhibited the action of sulphanilamide. Then it was found that pus, peptone, and products of tissue breakdown, would inhibit the action. For these reasons the local application of the sulphonamides to septic areas has not been quite so successful.

The following experiment illustrates the effect of streptococci in inhibiting the action of sulphanilamide. A large number of haemolytic streptococci, sensitive to sulphanilamide, were suspended in a 1 % solution of the drug and allowed to extract for an hour or two. They were then centrifuged out and the supernatant fluid was boiled to kill any remaining organisms. Serial dilutions of this

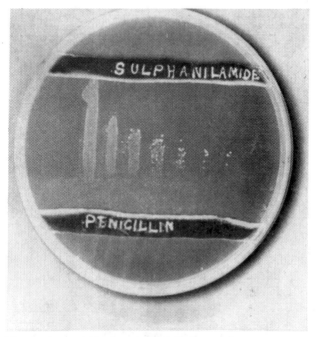

Plate I. Comparison of sensitivity of a haemolytic streptococcus to penicillin and sulphanilamide by the gutter method.

Dilutions of streptococci streaked between gutters containing penicillin and sulphanilamide. With penicillin there is little difference whatever the size of the inoculum. With sulphanilamide there is no inhibition of the undiluted culture.

[To face p. 26

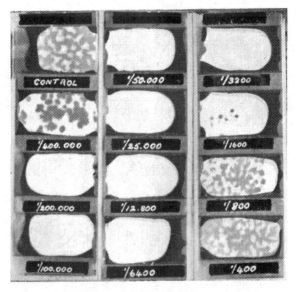

Plate II. Inhibition of sulphanilamide by streptococci.

Sulphanilamide 1 per cent. was treated with haemolytic streptococci (which were subsequently removed). It was then diluted with normal saline and mixed with an equal volume of human blood infected with haemolytic streptococci and grown in slide cells. The dark areas represent haemolysis due to growth of streptococci.

fluid were made and incubated with blood infected with a small number of the same haemolytic streptococci. (If the streptococci grew, the blood was haemolysed and served as an indicator.) In the strongest concentrations of the fluid the streptococci grew freely, but after it was diluted growth was completely inhibited, and this inhibition was manifest until the dilution reached 1 in 200,000 (Plate II). This was the dilution at which the original solution of sulphanilamide would have failed to inhibit if it had not been treated with streptococci.

The streptococci, therefore, produced something which did not destroy the sulphanilamide but merely inhibited its action.

This experiment furnishes an instance of a watery fluid which is not in itself antibacterial, but which becomes strongly bacteriostatic by the simple process of dilution with water.

Soon after the sulphonamides came into practice, also, it was discovered that some strains of what were generally sensitive microbes were resistant to their action. The result of widespread treatment was that the sensitive strains were largely displaced by insensitive strains. This was especially noticeable in gonococcal infections, and after a few years something like half of the gonococcal infections were sulphonamide insensitive.

27

This could be due to one of two things; the sensitive organisms might have been eliminated by treatment with the drug, while the insensitive ones persisted and were passed on from one individual to another; or that by insufficient treatment with the drug a sensitive microbe might have acquired a resistance or 'fastness' to the drug.

It is not difficult in the laboratory to make sensitive bacteria resistant to the sulphonamides, but this is not peculiar to the sulphonamides. There is probably no chemotherapeutic drug to which in suitable circumstances the bacteria cannot react by in some way acquiring 'fastness'.

In the first year of the war the sulphonamides had the field of chemotherapy of septic infections to themselves, but there were always the drawbacks I have mentioned. Later another type of sulphonamide, 'Marfanil', was introduced in Germany which for systemic administration had relatively little potency, but which was not inhibited by pus or the usual sulphonamide inhibitors. This was largely used in Germany throughout the war, but there is no doubt from what was seen in German hospitals when they were overrun that their methods of dealing with sepsis were far behind ours.

The sulphonamides did not directly kill the organisms—they stopped their growth, and the natural protective mechanisms of the body had to complete their destruction. This explained why in some cases of rather long-continued streptococcal septicaemia sulphanilamide failed to save the patient, although the *Streptococcus* was fully sensitive to the drug; the protective mechanism of the body—the opsonic power and phagocytes—had become worn out and failed.

Fildes introduced a most attractive theory of the action of chemotherapeutic drugs. It was that these drugs had a chemical structure so similar to an 'essential metabolite' of the sensitive organism that it deluded the organism into the belief that it was the essential metabolite. The organism therefore took it up, and then its receptors became filled with the drug so that it was unable to take up the essential metabolite which was necessary for its growth. Thus it was prevented from growing and died or was an easy prey for the body cells. This theory had been supported by many experimental facts and may give a most profitable guide to future advances in chemotherapy.

But another completely different type of chemotherapeutic drug appeared, namely, penicillin. This actually was described years before the sulphonamides appeared, but it was only concentrated sufficiently for practical chemotherapeutic use in 1940.

The story of penicillin has often been told in the last few years. How, in 1928, a mould spore contaminating one of my culture plates at St Mary's Hospital produced an effect which called for investigation; how I found that this mould—a *Penicillium*—made in its growth a diffusible and very selective antibacterial agent which I christened Penicillin; how this substance, unlike the older antiseptics, killed the bacteria but was non-toxic to animals or to human leucocytes; how I failed to concentrate this substance from lack of sufficient chemical assistance, so that it was only 10 years afterwards, when chemotherapy of septic infections was a predominant thought in the physician's mind, that Florey and his colleagues at Oxford embarked on a study of antibiotic substances, and succeeded in concentrating penicillin and showing its wonderful therapeutic properties; how this happened at a critical stage of the war, and how they took their information to America and induced the authorities there to produce penicillin on a large scale; how the Americans improved methods of production so that on D day there was enough penicillin for every wounded man who needed it, and how this result was obtained by the closest co-operation between Governments, industrialists, scientists and workmen on both sides of the Atlantic without thought of patents or other restrictive measures. Everyone had a near relative in the fighting line and there was the urge to help him, so progress and production went on at an unprecedented pace.

Penicillin is the most powerful chemotherapeutic drug yet introduced. Even when it is diluted 80,000,000 times it will still inhibit the growth of *Staphylococcus*. This is a formidable dilution, but the figure conveys little except a series of many naughts. Suppose we translate it into something concrete. If a drop of water is diluted 80,000,000 times it would fill over 6000 whisky bottles.

We have already seen that all the older antiseptics were more toxic to leucocytes than to bacteria. The sulphonamides were much more toxic to bacteria than to leucocytes, but they had some poisonous action on the whole human organism. Here in penicillin we had a substance extremely toxic to some bacteria but almost completely nontoxic to man. And it not only stopped the growth of the bacteria, it killed them, so it was effective even if the natural protective mechanism of the body was deficient. It was effective, too, in pus and in the presence of other substances which inhibited sulphonamide activity.

Penicillin has proved itself in war casualties and in a great variety of the ordinary civil illnesses, but it is specific, and there are many common infections on which it has no effect. Perhaps the most striking results have been in venereal disease. Gonococcal infections are eradicated with a single injection and syphilis in most cases by a treatment of under 10 days. Subacute bacterial endocarditis, too, was a disease which until recently was almost invariably fatal. Now with penicillin treatment there are something like 70% recoveries.

So far in this country penicillin has been under strict control, but soon it will be on sale in the chemists' shops. It is to be hoped that it will not be abused as were the sulphonamides. It is the only chemotherapeutic drug which has no toxic properties—in the ordinary sense of the word it is almost impossible to give an overdose—so there is no medical reason for underdosage. It is the administration of too small doses which leads to the production of resistant strains of bacteria, so the rule in penicillin treatment should be to give enough. If more than enough is given there is no harm to the patient but merely a little waste—but that is not serious when there is a plentiful supply.

But I am not giving you a discourse on penicillin. Suffice it to say that it has made medicine and surgery easier in many directions, and in the near future its merits will be proved in veterinary medicine and possibly in horticulture.

The spectacular success of penicillin has stimulated the most intensive research into other antibiotics in the hope of finding something as good or even better.

Gramicidin and Tyrothricin

But even before penicillin was publicized another antibiotic had been introduced by Dubos in 1939. This was a substance made by the *Bacillus brevis*, which had a very powerful inhibitory action on the Gram-positive bacteria. This substance was originally named gramicidin, but later the name was changed to tyrothricin, when it was found to be a mixture of two antibiotic substances—true gramicidin and tyrocidine. Gramicidin has proved to be a very useful local application to infected areas. It has an inhibitory power on bacteria far in excess of its antileucocytic power, but unfortunately it is toxic when injected, so that it cannot be used for systemic treatment. If penicillin had not appeared it is likely that gramicidin or tyrothricin would have been much more extensively used, but penicillin, which is quite non-toxic, can be used either locally or systemically for almost every condition which would be benefited by gramicidin.

Streptomycin

Waksman in 1943 described this antibiotic, which is produced by *Streptomyces griseus*. This substance has very little toxicity and has a powerful action on many of the Gram-negative organisms. It has been used in tularaemia, undulant fever, typhoid fever, and *B. coli* infections, but the greatest interest has been in its action on the tubercle bacillus. *In vitro* it has a very powerful inhibitory action on this bacillus, and in guinea-pigs it has been shown to have a definite curative action. In man, however, the clinical results have not been entirely successful, but in streptomycin we have a chemical which does have *in vivo* a definite action on the tubercle bacillus and which is relatively non-toxic. This is a great advance and may lead to startling results. One possible drawback may be that bacilli appear to acquire rapidly a fastness to streptomycin, much more rapidly than they do to penicillin or even the sulphonamides.

Many other antibiotics have been described in the last five years. Most of them are too toxic for use, but there are some which so far have promise in preliminary experiments. Whether they are going to be valuable chemotherapeutic agents belongs to the future.

Let us now consider the future. There are now certain definite lines on which research is proceeding in antibacterial chemotherapy.

Fildes's theory of the action of chemotherapeutic drugs has already led to certain results—not sufficiently powerful to have made wonderful advances in practical therapeutics—but the work goes on, and from it at any time some new antibacterial chemical combination may emerge. All this is dependent on further fundamental research on the essential metabolites necessary for the growth of different bacteria.

Bacteriologists and mycologists are, by more or less established methods, investigating all sorts of moulds and bacteria to see if they produce antibiotic substances. The chemist concentrates or purifies the active substance, and then the experimental pathologist tests the concentrate for activity and toxicity. There are teams of workers who are thus investigating every bacillus and every mould in the collections which exist in various countries. This is useful team work and may lead to something of practical importance, but it is reminiscent of the momentous German researches lacking in inspiration but which by sheer mass of labour bear some fruit. This plodding along appeals to many, but no one can expect the results to be revolutionary.

I have already mentioned some antibiotics which have given promise, and there are others which in preliminary experiments seem to have possibilities. It seems likely that in the next few years a combination of antibiotics with different antibacterial spectra will furnish a 'cribrum therapeuticum' from which fewer and fewer infecting bacteria will escape.

Then the work on antibiotics has led to the discovery of many new chemical combinations possessing antibacterial powers. Most of the antibiotics have certain disadvantages—many of them are too toxic—but it may not be beyond the powers of the organic chemists to alter the formula in such a way that the antibiotic power is retained, but the toxic power reduced to such an extent that these substances can be used therapeutically.

The most important chemotherapeutic want in Britain at the moment is a central institute for fundamental research in microbiology. In the past we have no reason to be ashamed of the results we have achieved in this direction, but the researches have been done in diverse institutions, often in the worker's spare time, and there have been times when the facilities for extending new discoveries did not exist. In Britain we are far behind the

United States and, indeed, some of the smaller countries of the Continent of Europe in this respect, and it seems to me very necessary that here we should have a complete institute comprising bacteriologists, mycologists, protozoologists, biologists, biochemists, organic chemists, experimental pathologists and pharmacologists. It would probably be a good investment as well as an advertisement for British biological science.

Take penicillin as an example. Discovered here in 1928 in a hospital bacteriological laboratory where the chemical facilities were lacking, then worked on in a biochemical laboratory where the bacteriological co-operation failed, it had to wait 10 years before it was concentrated sufficiently to show its remarkable chemotherapeutic properties. Even then there were difficulties in developing it in this country, with the result that the Americans have reaped a large part of the reward.

Had we had a microbiological institute such as I have envisaged, penicillin could have been developed here years ago, and this one substance could well have paid the cost of the institute over a long period of years, to say nothing of a certain amount of alleviation of suffering in the interim period. It is not too late to found such an institute. Enormous sums are being spent on national medical service—a large amount could well be spent on a national agricultural and veterinary research service, and we have unique association with the tropics in all matters. A small fraction of this money would found a microbiological institute which would, I am quite sure, pay handsome dividends in discoveries of importance in medicine, agriculture and industry. I am not the first to cry out for such an institute. The Royal Society's report on the needs of research in fundamental science after the war (issued in January 1945) makes the following recommendation:

'There is an urgent need for the establishment of an institute of general microbiology which should be the focal point for microbiological research in the Empire and should also have advisory and consultative functions.'

One misfortune is that it is nobody's baby. The Medical Research Council, the Agricultural Research Council and the Department of Scientific and Industrial Research, and other bodies may recognize the importance of such an institute, but as its activities spread over medicine, veterinary medicine, agriculture and industry, none of them feels justified in shouldering the burden.

With supertax so high there were possibilities of obtaining considerable sums of money for such an institute from the very rich under a seven-year covenant which allowed the institution to recover income tax and supertax. But I noticed the other day in the papers that a suggestion had been made in the House of Commons that steps would be taken to stop that 'racket'.

If far-sighted wealthy men are prevented from providing funds and if the Government will not provide funds there is no hope for any such an innovation as an institute for fundamental research in microbiology. Then we shall have to watch other more enlightened countries getting ahead and resign ourselves to be mere followers instead of leaders.

As to chemotherapeutic research in general I should like to conclude with a quotation from Mervyn Gordon: 'No research is ever quite complete. It is the glory of a good bit of work that it opens the way for something still better, and thus rapidly leads to its own eclipse. The object of research is the advancement, not of the investigator, but of knowledge.'

Printed in the United States
By Bookmasters